Striving for a cancer free tomorrow:
Uniting for a Healthier World"

BILLIE .R. FlORES

table of contents

Introduction:

Introduction:

Hope is a beacon of light in a world where the fight against cancer is still ongoing.

"Striving for a Cancer-Free Tomorrow" is more than just a book; it is a road map to a better, healthier future and a celebration of human fortitude.

Millions of people have been affected by the terrible adversary of cancer. It has been fought by scientists, caregivers, and survivors with unyielding tenacity.

This book's pages will take you on an enthralling trip through the victories of courageous people who faced cancer head-on and won.

Bravery, faith, and an unbreakable spirit that pave the way for a better future are the threads that connect their unique experiences.

However, this book also offers readers a glimpse into the cutting-edge world of research and invention in addition to personal stories.

Find more about the technical developments that are revolutionizing cancer prevention and treatment.

Discover the never-ending quest for knowledge that propels researchers to solve the puzzles surrounding this illness and bring us one step closer to a world free of cancer.

We kindly ask you to join us in "Striving for a Cancer-Free Tomorrow" as we work to build a more positive, healthy, and future.

It serves as a call to action for cooperation, a celebration of human creativity, and a warning that we can overcome even the most difficult obstacles when we work together.

Welcome to a future where we may create one page at a time and in which the fight against cancer joins hope, tenacity, and advancement.

Chapter 1:

1. Early signs of the "silent killer" include:

Two Early 'Silent Killer' Symptoms There Are Known Cases of Cancer

The death of US TV personality Jerry Springer has recently attracted attention to pancreatic cancer, which is frequently referred to as a "silent killer" due to its difficult-to-detect early-stage symptoms.

Only 5% of those who have the disease survive for more than ten years after diagnosis, making it one of the cancers with the lowest survival rates overall.

However, two new warning indicators that can aid medical professionals in diagnosing cancer have been discovered owing to research at the Nuffield Department of Primary Health Care Sciences.

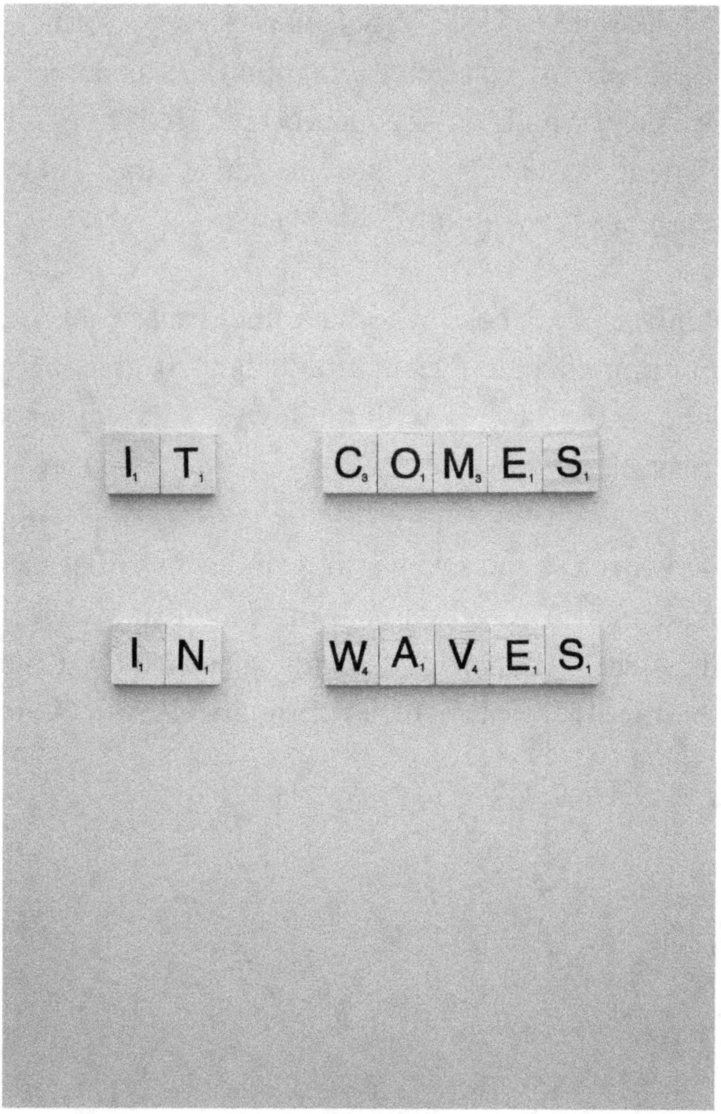

IT COMES

IN WAVES

Treatment Pancreatic Cancer Early Warning Signs

Up until recently, we were aware that pancreatic cancer's primary symptoms included jaundice, loss of appetite or unintended weight loss, fatigue or a lack of vitality, and a high fever or a hot, shaky feeling.

There are now two symptoms that can show up to a year before a diagnosis. Increased thirst and dark yellow urine are two of these.

Despite the fact that these symptoms may not be a sign of pancreatic cancer, researchers discovered that those who had the disease had a higher likelihood of exhibiting them up to a year before their diagnosis.

This is incredibly encouraging news for the future of pancreatic cancer treatment, and Dr. Wiqi Liao from the Nuffield Department of Primary Health Care Sciences is optimistic that

GPs will now be more aware and confident in referring patients for urgent tests. He declared:

"These new findings allow us to continue our investigation into the warning signs and symptoms of pancreatic cancer. This will make it simpler for physicians to select people for urgent testing, particularly when those patients present with a multitude of hazy symptoms.

- individuals who acquire pancreatic cancer.

Over half of all diagnoses of pancreatic cancer in adults are over the age of 75, whereas cases in people under the age of 40 are quite uncommon, according to Cancer Research UK. However, there are some factors that may increase your risk of contracting the sickness, such as:

Obesity is a factor in more than 10% of pancreatic cancer cases.

About 20% of instances include people who smoke or use smokeless tobacco, such as cigarettes, cigars, pipes, and chewing tobacco.

Genetic factors account for 5–10% of cases.

What to Do If You Think You May Have Pancreatic Cancer?
If you have jaundice, have had diarrhea for more than seven days, have been vomiting for more than two days, or are having other symptoms that worry you, the NHS advice dial 111 for advice.

However, if you've dropped a large amount of weight, you should see a doctor.

over the past six to twelve months without attempting it, have additional pancreatic cancer symptoms that don't go away after two weeks, or have a condition that causes digestive symptoms that don't go away after two weeks of using your standard treatments.

The NHS also emphasizes the importance of seeing a GP about these symptoms even though they can potentially be signs of a variety of other disorders and don't necessarily indicate cancer.

2.The Cancer Mysteries

Millions of people around the world have been impacted by cancer disease.

It is a complicated condition that can develop as a result of a confluence of hereditary and environmental variables.

Although the exact cause of cancer is still unknown, it is known that when cells in our bodies divide and develop in an uncontrolled way, a lump of tissue known as a tumor results.

While some tumors are benign and do not spread to other body areas, others are malignant and have the potential to do so, potentially posing major health risks.

- Cancer: Is it genetic?

A complicated illness like cancer may develop as a result of both hereditary and environmental causes. There is evidence that some cancers can run in families, indicating that the illness might have a genetic component.

However, genetics alone is not to blame for the majority of cancer instances. Instead, a person's chance of developing cancer can be increased by a mix of hereditary and environmental variables, including exposure to specific chemicals and lifestyle decisions.

- What are some typical cancer causes?

Numerous elements, such as the following, can raise someone's risk of getting cancer:

exposure to particular chemicals and materials
unhealthy eating habits and inactivity
alcohol and tobacco use

infection with specific contagions, similar as hepatitis B and C and the mortal papillomavirus(HPV), radioactive impurity family cancer history Why Does Cancer Affect Some People But Not Others? Why some people get cancer while others don't isn't completely understood.

Still, it's believed that a person's chance of acquiring cancer can be increased by a blend of heritable and environmental factors, including exposure to specific chemicals and life choices.

It's pivotal to realize that indeed if a person has a high threat of acquiring cancer, the complaint doesn't inescapably follow.

Understanding Men's and Women's Cancer While both men and women can develop cancer, some cancers are more common in one gender than the other. For example, men are more likely to develop prostate cancer than women are to develop bone cancer.

But it's pivotal to realize that cancer can strike anyone, anyhow of gender. Are There Any Symptoms or Signs to Fete Bone Cancer in its Early Stages?

Bone cancer may not show any signs in its early stages. still, when the illness worsens, the following symptoms could crop constantly bone or underarm thickening or a lump revision in the bone's size or form Blunt discharge

alterations to the breast's skin, such as dimpling or puckering
flipped nipple

It is crucial to remember that these symptoms are not invariably a sign of breast cancer and may potentially be brought on by other illnesses. If you notice any changes in your breasts, it's crucial to consult a doctor.

How Is Cancer Found Out? What Kinds of Screening Techniques Are There?

There are several screening techniques that can be used to find cancer, including:

- Examination of the body

a blood test
Radiology procedures like X-rays, CT scans, and MRIs
Performing a biopsy, which entails taking a sample of tissue from the injured area to be examined

The optimal screening techniques for your particular needs should be discussed with a doctor, as early discovery is essential for effective treatment.

- The Stages of Cancer

Typically, cancer is divided into four stages, with stage 0 denoting the disease's earliest stage and stage IV denoting the most advanced state. The progression and spread of the disease, as well as the most effective course of therapy, are determined by the stages of cancer.

Stage 0:

This is the earliest stage of cancer, which denotes that the cancer cells have not yet spread to other places of the body and are only present where they first manifested.

Phase I:

While the cancer cells are still regarded as confined and have not moved to distant parts of the body at this stage, they have begun to invade neighboring tissues and organs.

2nd stage:

At this point, the cancer has likely migrated to the lymph nodes and has already begun to affect the tissues and organs surrounding.

stage three

At this point, the cancer has likely progressed to the lymph nodes and to other far-flung areas of the body.

stage four:

This is the most advanced stage of cancer, and it indicates that the disease has gone to the bones, liver, lungs, or brain, among other organs.

Cancer is a set of complicated, varied illnesses that can manifest and advance differently for every patient.

The phases of cancer are crucial for choosing the appropriate course of therapy and for educating patients and medical professionals about the development and spread of the illness.

Chapter 2:

1. Enhancing the Defenses in Your Body:

Perhaps you've seen or read about products that promise to "boost" your immune system. What does that actually mean, and is that even the proper objective?

Our bodies don't have a single immune system, despite common perception. According to Cara Anselmo, a clinical dietitian nutritionist at Memorial Sloan Kettering Cancer Center, the immune system is actually made up of numerous organs, cells, and proteins that cooperate to ward off illnesses.

Some cancer therapies might decrease an individual's immune system, making it difficult for their body to effectively fight against infection.

But even for them, according to Ms. Anselmo, the objective is not to accelerate quickly. Whether you have cancer or not, it's important to maintain a healthy balance in your immune system.

Maintaining healthy behaviors will keep your body's systems running smoothly. Wintertime is a crucial time because germs are more likely to spread inside.

Think of the phrase "immune system" as being replaced with "a healthy body," advises Ms. Anselmo. Here are some of her tips for boosting your resistance.

- Organize your plate.

There is no one magic food that will keep your immunity in check, just as there is no one element to the immune system (sorry!).

Still, a lot of foods can be salutary. Everyone has heard how vitamin C works to fight off conditions like snap.

There are several reasons why this vitamin deserves special citation. Since vitamin C is an antioxidant, it counteracts the destructive, cell-destroying chemicals known as free revolutionaries. Also, it promotes the development of antibodies and white blood cells, both of which work to fight infection. Vitamin C can not be produced by the body; it's only set up in foods.

Still, that doesn't obligate you to consume one orange each day. In addition, foods like tomatoes, bell peppers, and strawberries, to mention a many, contain vitaminC.

Although consuming foods high in vitamin C is necessary, most people do not need to take vitamin C supplements.

Multitudinous other nutrients help maintain a strong vulnerable system. Systemic inflammation can be dropped by eating a diet high in cruciferous vegetables, similar as broccoli, cauliflower, kale, and Brussels sprouts.

The Anti-inflammatory parcels of allium vegetables including garlic, scallions, and onion are analogous. The nutritive content of these particulars is the same whether you eat them cooked or raw. Protein is also pivotal.

Proteins from both creatures and shops are used to produce new cells and form damaged towels, acting as a descent and protective armament against overrunning organisms.

2. Drink plenty of water. " People concentrate on food so much, and food is important, but our

mucus membranes are one line of defense against infection," To perform at their optimum, water keeps them wettish.

These shielding liners may be set up in your nose, mouth, and eyes, and they serve as bouncers at a club to keep out interferers. Still, did you know that some body corridors, including the stomach and the womanish and manly reproductive systems, have mucous membranes covering them as well?

The advice to consume eight spectacles of water each day may not be necessary. You can get technical advice from your professional dietitian or nutritionist.

3. Avoid depending on supplements.
They are not intended to replace a balanced diet. However, consult your medical team before taking any supplements because some of them, like vitamin D (more on that later), can prevent or remedy some nutritional deficits.

Just remember to not conflate "natural" and "safe." "Those promoted for 'boosting immunity,'" adds Ms. Anselmo, "can do more harm than good." This is true of any oral vitamin, mineral, herbal, or other supplements.

4. corroborate your vitamin D input. There's no distrustfulness about it. It helps ameliorate strength.

But vitamin D also maintains the health of T cells and macrophages, two types of cells that fight complaints.

Humans gain this mineral by exposure to the sun rather than through eating. " You could eat the healthiest diet in the world and still not get enough vitamin D,"Ms.

Anselmo asserts. Indeed milk, which we've each been told is an awful source, is inadequate. You could bear a supplement because numerous people are unfortunately vitamin D deficient due to the long, chilly layoffs.

Your situations can be examined by your croaker through a blood test.

5. Continue going. Your lungs and airways can come free of microorganisms if you exercise. Also, it reduces the release of stress hormones, which is important as too important stress might vitiate impunity.

You do not have to put forth a lot of trouble to get the prices. Walking is a tone- paced exertion that does not bear any special outfit, according toMs.

Anselmo. She also suggests doing exercises that increase your strength, like yoga or lifting weights.

Anselmo gives the following guidance once your croaker
has given the go- ahead to begin a new drill authority" hear to your body, start laggardly, and increase the intensity and frequency gradually."

6. Make sleep a precedent. We constantly believe that we can go without sleep if we follow a healthy diet and exercise authority. But sleep is actually relatively important.

The vulnerable system is laboriously releasing proteins that bolster the body's viral defenses while we sleep.

She advises that taking day naps to catch up is fine, but try to limit them to no further than 30 twinkles to avoid changing your circadian cycle.

Chapter 3:

1. Our secret weapon is food.

Our secret weapon is food. Food can provide our bodies with everything they require to thrive, whether we're running a marathon or taking a day off.

Our body is metabolically active even while we are at rest. Our digestive system, liver, heart, lungs, kidneys, muscles, brain, central nervous system, liver, and muscles all operate around the clock to keep us alive.

That much labor requires energy. Daily tasks and exercise might contribute 20% to 250% more energy requirements than what our body needs at rest.

Eating from a variety of food groups is necessary to maintain a balanced intake. There are more than 40 nutrients required for growth, and neither a single food nor a dietary group can supply all of them.

Because nutrients complement one another, eating too much of one can alter how efficiently our body uses another.

We could become so preoccupied with a single objective, such as muscular growth, that we lose sight of all the other critical activities that are constantly taking place.

To maintain balance, one must consume enough to support activity and performance goals. Many people eat more than they need, but those who are really active and work out for at least 60 minutes a day frequently struggle to consume enough calories to meet their essential physiological needs.

When you are properly fuelled, you should feel full and enthusiastic rather than ravenous and cranky.

Food quality is also important; stay near to the farm. Highly processed foods frequently lack vital nutrients or contain extra substances that interfere with the balance of all our vital systems.

Eat complete foods and foods with naturally existing nutrients to ensure that you are giving your body the high-quality nourishment it needs.

The time of your meal also counts. While eating at least three times a day is a good place to start, not eating for an extended period of time can disrupt homeostasis.

To maximize the benefits of a workout session, timing is also crucial.

Eating before and immediately after a strenuous or prolonged workout will ensure that it is of the highest quality, restore any fuel that has been used, and start the repair, recovery, and synthesis of new muscle tissue.

the human performance optimization educational division of the Consortium for Health and Military Performance, a Department of Defense Center of Excellence situated at the Uniformed Services University, for further details on nutrition for activity and performance.

All the components of Total Force fitness are supported by HPRC's comprehensive, performance-optimization services, which assist military personnel in remaining resilient, appropriately fueled and hydrated, socially connected, and physically and psychologically fit.

2. Cancer Treatment: Using Your Own Immune System

Cancer Treatment: Using Your Own Immune System

Your body's immune system defends itself against infections.

Your immune system is stimulated through immunotherapy, a type of medical therapy, to help fight cancer.

Your body has a variety of immune cell types. Various cells combat various forms of cancer.

For instance, the immune system uses T cells, a particular type of white blood cell, to combat cancer:
• Cancer is perceived by T cells as "foreign" tissue that doesn't belong in the body.
• Once the cancer cells have been eliminated, an immune system "checkpoint" prevents the T cells from continuing to assault the cancer cells. It safeguards healthy cells.

Cancer cells may deceive the immune system into believing they are healthy cells. This is one way in which cancer can sometimes outsmart the immune system.

The "checkpoint" process may be activated by cancer cells. This may cause the immune system to prematurely halt its battle on the malignancy.

• How immunotherapy for cancer operates
There are now three main categories of immunotherapy:
Immune checkpoint blockadeIn this method, medications are used to halt the "checkpoint" procedure.

This enables the T cells to continue battling malignancy.
There are now a number of checkpoint inhibitor medications that have received FDA approval. Yervoy®, Keytruda®, and Opdivo® are a few examples of the brand names.

individual cell treatment
With this method, the body's immune cells are modified to improve their capacity to combat cancer.

There are two strategies to accomplish this: • By boosting immune system cell numbers to the point where they outnumber cancer cells.

• By altering the immune cells' genetic composition.

This may cause the immune system to target particular cancer types.

• CAR T cell therapy is one of the current forms of individualized cell treatment in use.

- vaccines for cancer

Researchers are working on vaccines that could instruct the immune system to spot and kill cancer before it spreads or reappears.

Long after the original cancer has faded, it constantly spreads to other body corridors or comes back.

This new strategy suggests that vaccines may be suitable to fete before cases of cancer and launch the proper vulnerable response when it reappears.

The development of vaccinations against colorful excrescences is continuously being pursued by experimenters.

sometimes, further than one immunotherapy modality or immunotherapy drug will be administered coincidently. Along with chemotherapy and radiation, immunotherapy is an option.

This could ameliorate the efficacy of conventional cancer treatments. The immunotherapy system developed at Stony Brook One of the most recent developments in cancer treatment is immunotherapy.

Everybody formerly has a vulnerable system that defends them from illnesses. However, everyone wins, If we can boost the vulnerable system to fight cancer.

We seek to find curatives that can significantly ameliorate the lives of the individualities we serve in Suffolk and Nassau Counties.

We want to ameliorate the effectiveness, comfort, and convenience of cancer treatment for our cases.

Our clinical trial program for cancer immunotherapy is likewise relatively active. Cases can bestow to share in clinical studies where new immunotherapy curatives are being tested on them. To learn further about cancer immunotherapy or to enquire about a study,

Chapter 4:

1.Cancer and physical activity

Cancer and physical activity
Thankfully, our bodies still have mechanisms in place to combat the ability of these cancer cells to survive.

It is well known that cancer cells do not function effectively in the presence of oxygen since cancer is commonly recognized as a disease of metabolic dysregulation (see the explanation above).

Right, that's a simple solution—just saturate cancer cells with oxygen, and they will perish. Yes, but getting the oxygen inside the cancer cell is the difficult part.

Numerous complementary and alternative cancer treatments can successfully produce this advantageous environment and deliver oxygen to a cancer cell's inner core.

This explains why treatments like high-dose vitamin C and DCA therapy are so effective in the therapeutic setting.

Even if these treatments are effective, it is difficult to continuously provide all cancer cells with oxygen (24 hours a day, 7 days a week). This is where the advantages of physical activity are so helpful and practical!

So, what must I do, and how precisely does this operate?

The body requires extra oxygen when participating in any type of lengthy physical exercise, even if it only lasts for 15 minutes at a time (you need more oxygen to keep those muscles working!).

By being active, the body provides oxygen to every cell, including cancer cells, allowing mitochondria to produce the necessary energy. However, cancer cells dislike this.

Cancer cells basically put their mitochondria to "sleep" in order to survive, preventing the production of aerobic energy (energy from oxygen) when there is oxygen present.

However, cancer cells' mitochondria become more 'alive' the more oxygen that is supplied to the cells.

The stress of being in the presence of oxygen shifts cancer cells' energy production away from anaerobic (lactic acid) energy creation to that of aerobic energy creation, ultimately leading to the death of the cancer cell.

Therefore, as our bodies use more oxygen, it becomes less conducive to cancer surviving, growing, and disseminating (and no, increased blood inflow, oxygen, and nutrition rotation with ever- adding oxygen doesn't feed cancer cells or beget them to circulate; this concern has been completely disproven and put to rest).

The stylish terrain to fight cancer can be created by engaging in physical exercise. All that's truly needed are brief(15 nanosecond) bursts of focused exertion performed at least 1- 2 times per day and 3 – 4 times(minimum) per week.

The share will be fully filled with brisk walking, a quick jam, or a hike to start reaping the advantages.

Exercise is an element of a comprehensive approach to cancer care that Cornerstone NaturopathicInc. uses.

can help with. Start your integrative cancer care authority right down if you want to do yourself a favor.

Both the probability of developing cancer and the side goods of cancer treatments are reduced by physical exertion.

Also, it improves the health of cases and the prognosis for those who have cancer.

" Before, it was allowed that after a cancer opinion, people should just rest. At the moment, there's growing scientific evidence that exercise may indeed ameliorate a cancer case's prognosis.

Still, Tiia Koivula, an exploration adjunct, explains that the processes through which exercise exerts control over cancer aren't yet completely known.

The 10-minute drill was sufficient.

28 recently diagnosed carcinoma and bone cancer cases were included in the two studies.

Cases with carcinoma ranged in age from 20 to 69, whereas those with bone cancer ranged in age from 37 to 73.

The actors engaged in a 10- nanosecond cycling exertion each day of the study. Two times ahead and two times after the drill, blood samples were taken.

According to Koivula, each case's pedal resistance was customized to correspond to either mild or moderate physical exertion.

The main idea was for cases to bike continuously for 10 twinkles without getting exhausted and to increase their heart rate at the same time.

The experimenters measured the attention of colorful vulnerable cells,
often known as leukocytes or white blood cells,
in the blood samples.

They compared the cell counts in the samples taken ahead and after the exercise. The amount of vulnerable cells suitable to annihilate cancer cells rose after exercise. Cases with melanoma endured an increase in cytotoxic 'I' cells and natural killer cells throughout the drill.

Physical exercise increased the total number of leukocytes as well as the volume of intermediate monocytes, B cells, cytotoxic T cells, and natural killer cells in bone cancer cases.

Immune cell counts for the maturity of cases snappily and curtly regressed to birth situations as seen in blood samples taken 30 beats after exercise.

The observed increase in cytotoxic vulnerable cells during exercise in both patient populations was particularly intriguing. According to Koivula, these vulnerable cells have the power to count cancer cells.

The amount of physical exertion and the change in vulnerable cell numbers in both patient groups were also linked, the researchers set up. further vulnerable cells were circulated into the body when the cases' heart rate and blood pressure increased."

Our results illuminate that indeed light or moderate intensity exercise lasting just 10 beats can elevate the count of vital vulnerable cells involved in combating cancer, despite indicating that lower exercise intensity leads to increased transfer of vulnerable cells from storage organs to the bloodstream,"

1. Workout as Defense

Cancer risk is decreased with regular exercise. Similarly, sitting and inactivity can raise your risk of getting cancer.

According to studies, maintaining a healthy weight, getting enough exercise, and eating well helps prevent at least one-third of the most frequent malignancies.

The finest thing you can do for yourself is regular exercise. Do your chores around the house on a bicycle, use the stairs instead of the elevator, and avoid driving. Everything, including brief exercise sessions, benefits your health.

It is better to choose regular, healthy exercise over sporadic trips to the gym. However, frequent, demanding fitness training is the most efficient strategy to lower the risk of cancer from a cancer prevention perspective.

Even yet, leading a sedentary lifestyle negates the protective effects of exercise on health issues.

- Which forms of cancer can exercise prevent?

Bowel, breast, and uterine cancer are all prevented by exercise.

Your risk of developing cancer decreases with increased exercise. The more physically taxing the exercise, the more effectively it lowers the risk of cancer.

Exercise should be consistent (ideally daily, at least five times a week), prolonged (through your entire life), and moderate to heavy.

When compared to exercising the least, a minimum of seven hours per week reduces the risk of breast cancer by 25%.

When compared to people who don't exercise, the risk of colon cancer is roughly 25% lower in regular exercisers, and up to 40% lower in some studies.

Your risk of developing cancer decreases the more you exercise.

Uterine cancer risk rises with adult weight gain, especially around the waist.

The greater the amount of excess weight, the higher the cancer risk. Heavy or difficult exercise can cut the risk of uterine cancer by up to 40%, especially in obese women.

Additionally, exercise aids in controlling weight. You can further lower your chances of breast cancer and colon cancer by maintaining a healthy weight.

Additionally, keeping a healthy weight may help lower your chance of developing

several other cancers, including oesophageal, pancreatic, and kidney cancer.

Chapter 5:

1. Mind Over Matter

The power of study sorely, there's little evidence that stations can change the course of cancer's natural history, despite the fact that the power of the mind is only now starting to be understood.

The presence of church and religion as well as a strong social support network, still, appear to be constant factors in conserving a high quality of life in those with advanced cancer.

People who have many or no social connections have a mainly advanced mortality rate than those who have strong social ties to musketeers and family.

Being wedded is good for your health, whereas being widowed is bad for your health, especially if you are a man.

It's probable that this sense of closeness serves as a predictor of those who cleave rigorously to prescribed medical procedures and who lead a healthy life in terms of eating, rest, and exercise.

Are there any connections between this and cancer cases?

It could. According to one study, bone cancer cases of all races had lower survival rates when they demanded intimate connections and access to emotional support.

According to a different study, cases' perceived lack of social support was linked to a decline in supplemental blood NK cell exertion.

Naturally, no bone
has proven that NO exertion in supplemental blood is a predictor of any cancer- related outgrowth.

At least three randomized studies have demonstrated that cases with metastatic bone cancer, nasty carcinoma, or hematologic malice who were assigned to probative internal group treatment fared better than those who weren't enrolled in such a program.

In each of these explorations, the benefits of the intervention were notable, not subtle;

chemotherapeutic studies are infrequently as salutary as these cerebral support curatives feel to be.

still, it does not feel that there's any typical cerebral or personality profile that distinguishes the case who's more likely to survive for a long time.

Another element that has been proposed as a predictor of survival in cancer cases is church.

It's egregious that this element is delicate to quantify. The" death- bed conversion" is such a current circumstance that it has been made fun of and is now a cliché.

Fields was asked what he was doing because he wasn't known as a religious man when he was discovered by a friend flipping through the Bible in the midst of his terminal sickness.

He reportedly replied," Looking for loopholes," when asked what he was doing. Still, religious persuasions are immaculately suited to help people manage terminal complaints.

Does it count if someone has only lately joined a church or has attended for their entire life? Fresh exploration is needed in this area.

Creagan comes to the conclusion that among cancer cases, the biology of the illness is the primary predictor of survival, but that psychosocial and spiritual variables may affect quality of life and maybe indeed survival in some cases.

1. Stress-Proofing Your Life:

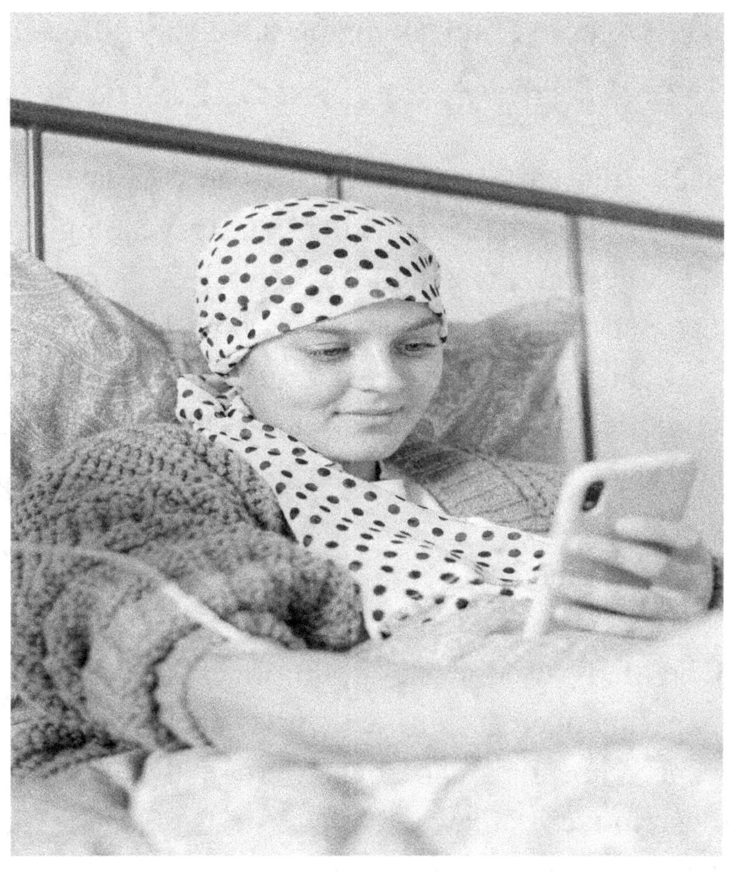

Cancer affects many aspects of a person's life, necessitating a comprehensive approach to therapy.

Studies utilizing combined medical and psychological therapies (MPIs), however, are few and far between. Poor quality of life (QoL) and excessive stress might adversely affect a patient's prognosis.

Thus, the study's objective was to evaluate the effects of combined medical and psychological therapies on stress and quality of life in cancer patients with head and neck, breast, and lung malignancies. These interventions included cognitive therapy, relaxation technique-guided imagery, and psychoeducation.

- Methods:

The study used a one-group pretest-posttest-pre experimental design and was carried out in cancer hospitals. The data were analyzed using descriptive statistics, paired t-tests, Cohen's d, and bar graphs.

- Results:

The combined MPIs had a significant influence on reducing overall stress as well as its numerous components, including fear, psychosomatic problems, knowledge deficiency, and constraints on daily activities.

Along with functional and symptom scores, significant changes were also observed in QoL and its domains, including global health status. The results revealed a large decline in the symptoms of fatigue, discomfort, insomnia, appetite loss, diarrhea, and constipation. However, there was a considerable improvement in the symptoms of physical, role, and emotional functioning.

- Conclusions:

It is clear that combining MPI benefits cancer patients by reducing stress and enhancing QoL, which can further improve their prognosis.

Chapter 6:

Early investigators

Mammograms and physical examinations are used in the conventional method of breast cancer screening.

Early cancer detection, which is essential for successful therapy, is difficult to achieve with these approaches.

I wanted to create a test that looked at people's DNA to see if particular genes were "turned off."

Basically, my goal was to create a rapid and simple test to identify cancer-causing mutations.

These are mutations, but not in the conventional sense of changing the sequence of a gene; rather, they alter how a gene is read:

Chromosomes would be the chapters, genes would be the sentences, and the individual letters would be the DNA if you were to imagine a genome as a book.

The typical mutations I was interested in would white out the entire phrase (gene) while leaving the actual words unaltered, but the traditional mutations would modify part of the words in each sentence, rendering it incomprehensible.

I used electrochemical techniques to find this. I was able to change DNA so that mutant forms would bind to an electrode surface more quickly.

I was able to gauge how difficult it was to conduct electricity to the solution at the electrode surface.

I would expect to see a greater resistance since the altered DNA bonded to the electrode surface more quickly.

I was able to distinguish between DNA that had been modified and DNA that was not. This difference in "resistance value"

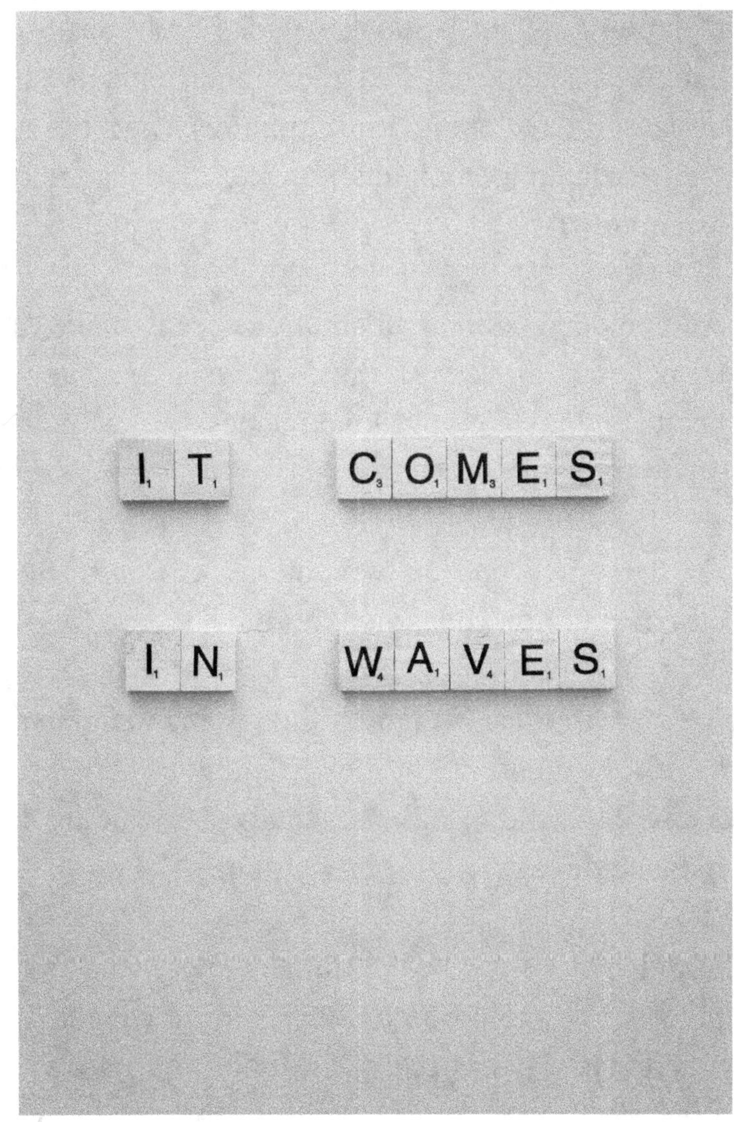

IT
COMES
IN
WAVES

Defending Against Shock Attacks Eight healthy habits can help you feel more and reduce your threat of developing multitudinous cancers, as well as heart complaints, stroke, diabetes, and osteoporosis.

And indeed minor adaptations can make a tremendous difference. thus, take charge of your health and inspire your loved bones
to do the same.

To start, pick one or two actions. Go on to the others after you've learned those.

1. Keep an Ideal Weight Although maintaining a healthy weight might be grueling , there are many fantastic health advantages, including a reduced threat of 13 different malice.

Simple advice can be helpful.However, your first precedence should be to stop gaining weight, If you're fat. This is really profitable on its own. When you are ready, aim to lose a lot of redundant pounds for an indeed larger enhancement in your health.

Tips Every day, include movement and physical exertion into your life.

Try to spend less time sitting in front of the television and computer, and stand further.

Consume plenitude of fruits, veggies, and whole grains in your diet. Eat more sluggishly, avoid sticky drinks, and choose lower servings.

2. Regular exercise There are many effects as healthy as regular physical exertion. Indeed though it's not always simple to find the time, it's pivotal to schedule at least 30 twinkles of exercise each day. Any volume is preferable than none, while further is indeed better. Tips: Pick pastimes you enjoy. Exercise can have numerous different effects, like cotillion , gardening, and walking.

By allowing the same quantum of time each day for exercise, you can make it a habit. Visit the spa during lunch or go for a perambulation after regale.

Exercise with a mate to make it pleasurable and maintain provocation. Go to the demesne, go on walks, and play energetic games as a family to stay active.

3. Avoid Smoking And Smokeless Tobacco Use

Along with other major issues, smoking leads to multitudinous cancers. So refrain from smoking.

Quitting is one of the finest effects you can do for your health if you bomb or use smokeless tobacco(similar to biting tobacco, snuff, or snus).

True, it's grueling , but you can do it! Tips Try again! Before you eventually give up, it constantly takes a lot of attempts.

Consult a croaker
about quitting, which can increase your odds of
success by two.

For backing, telephone 800- QUIT- Here and
now(866-shut- YES in Illinois) or go to
smokefree.gov. bandy the pitfalls of smoking,
vaping, and using smokeless tobacco with your
children.

The stylish way to impact children is by not
using tobacco yourself.

4. Consume a Balanced Diet Simple rules apply
to good eating in general. Keep red meat and
reused meat to a minimum and place a lesser
emphasis on fruits, vegetables, and healthy
grains. Also, it's pivotal to consume lower
unhealthy fats(impregnated and trans fats) while
consuming further polyunsaturated and
monounsaturated fats.

Tips Include fruits and vegetables in each mess. Fruit can be added to cereal. Veggies are a healthy snack.

Red and reused meat should be substituted with funk, fish, or legumes. rather of sticky cereal and white chuck
choose whole- grain druthers.

Pick dishes that are prepared with healthy fats like olive or canola oil painting. Reduce your consumption of store- bought snacks like eyefuls and fast food.

The stylish option is to eat a balanced diet, but if you constantly fall suddenly, suppose about taking a multivitamin.

5. Drink in Moderation- Zero Is Stylish Six different forms of cancer are more likely to do in people who drink alcohol. And as little as one drink a day can raise your threat of developing bone and colon cancer. In general, abstaining from alcohol is the healthiest option, while

moderate consumption may profit aged persons' hearts.

Tips Aim to drink alcohol-free potables at reflections and gatherings. Avoid gatherings where alcohol is served.

still, consult a healthcare provider, If you believe you have an alcohol use complaint. When applicable, talk to them about the pitfalls of alcohol and medicines.

6. Use sun protection measures and stay down from tanning beds While reposing in the warm sun can be pleasurable, inordinate sun exposure can beget skin cancer, including carcinoma.

Also, tanning beds have an analogous threat. Early skin damage in youths makes kid protection all the more pivotal.

Tips Avoid direct sun as much as you can between the hours of 10 am and 4 pm(high scorching hours).

The topmost way to defend yourself is to do this. Consider wearing headdresses, long sleeves, and sunscreen with an SPF of 30 or advanced.

Avoid using tanning beds or cells. cover children first, and also set a good illustration by constantly slipping sunscreen and applicable vesture.

7. Defend Yourself Against Sexually Transmitted conditions multitudinous malice can be brought on by sexually transmitted ails like the mortal papillomavirus(HPV), hepatitis, and HIV. Taking preventives to avoid certain ails can reduce the threat. Try to constantly engage in safer sexual geste
to reduce your threat of contracting an STD.

The advice for both grown-ups and children to get their HPV immunization is pivotal. In order to help prevent cancer in later life, boys and girls should both be vaccinated between the periods of 9 and 12. Still, the vaccine can be administered up to age 45 and is advised up to age 26.

For further information, consult your healthcare guru or go tocdc.gov/ HPV. Tips: Make sure your youth has the HPV vaccine as part of their routine vaccines from their doctor.

However, request it, If not. Speak to a provider about getting the HPV vaccine if you are a grown-up who hasn't formerly. Ask your parents or look for a dupe of your vaccination record if you are doubtful if you've had the vaccine. For further information about healthier coitus and safer coitus, go tocdc.gov/ sexualhealth. When applicable, talk to kids about the value of safe coitus and sexual responsibility.

8. Schedule wireworks There are several significant webbing examinations that can prop in cancer forestallment.

While some of these tests can help prevent cancer from being in the first place, others can help discover cancer beforehand, when it's further curable.

Consult your healthcare professional about screening at these periods; recommendations can change.

Chapter 7 :

1. cancer analysis

There is no illness or condition that can be more challenging for people to manage or survive than cancer.

The severity of cancer and the sheer number of individuals it affects make it the most widely conducted medical study worldwide.

Cancer scares people because it seems to be able to affect practically everyone.

Medical research is presently the best strategy to combat cancer.

Numerous medical researchers are working to develop a means of lowering or completely eliminating cancer.

It's not a simple undertaking, given the wide range of malignancies there are and their various causes.

Giving to cancer research is a fantastic approach to combat this terrible disease.

- What Exactly Does Cancer Research Do?

Many people assume that when they hear the term "cancer research" that everything is being done to discover a cure.

However, the truth is that there are numerous varieties of cancer research, and they all complement one another to either treat the illness or enhance people's quality of life. There are four categories of research:

The majority of individuals picture basic research when they think of cancer research.

Researchers try to comprehend the principles and basic features of how cancer behaves and responds in the body.

This research serves as the foundation for future efforts to prevent or treat cancer.

After basic research, clinical research is the next phase. Clinical research will attempt to develop and test new cancer-fighting medications and other technologies.

- This study also looks at every facet of patient care.

Research on the population focuses on identifying statistical patterns that can be used to pinpoint the origins of cancer.

Numerous cancers appear to occur at random. But study has greatly helped in foreseeing these changes.

Research on populations keeps track of care delivery and outcomes across multiple geographies.

Research that translates theoretical findings into practical applications is known as translational research.

Hospitals and clinics need to receive cancer research on patient care. The application of new methods will be aided through translational research.

1. using cutting-edge technologies in cancer research

Researchers and scientists have been searching for a cancer cure for hundreds of years, achieving incredible advancements in treatment along the way.

Expanded clinical trials have aided in the development of alternatives to chemotherapy for cancer patients and the exploration of the potential of precision medicine.

The infographic below, produced by Maryville University's online Master of Health Administration, provides more information regarding advancements in cancer therapy.

- Improvements to Clinical Trials

Clinical trials are performed to evaluate the outcomes of a newly created medication, medical procedure, or behavioral intervention.

- Clinical Trials in Modern History

The Pure Food and Drug Act, which was enacted in 1906 by President Theodore Roosevelt, forbade the selling of goods for purposes not specified on their labels. Decades later,

in 1962, the Kefauver-Harris Drug Amendment mandated that drug makers reveal accurate information about probable adverse effects and give proof of the efficacy of their products prior to approval.

Multicenter studies first appeared in 1944, allowing for a greater number of participants and a wider variety of population groups to be researched. This improved research trial designs and analysis.

Thirty years later, President Richard Nixon authorized the National Research Act, which mandated the approval of all human subjects research by an institutional review board.

Informed permission, the lack of coercion, properly designed scientific testing, and goodwill toward experiment subjects were all prerequisites for clinical trials set down by the Nuremberg Code in 1947.

The Nuremberg Code's ten ethical principles for human experimentation were supplemented in 1964 with the Helsinki Declaration, which added respect for the subject, the subject's right to self-determination, and the subject's freedom to make an informed choice about participating in research.

The U.S. Food and Drug Administration (FDA) published advice in 2019 that widened the eligibility requirements for cancer clinical trials to include more older persons.

The FDA believes that patients with terminal cancers should be eligible to participate in oncology clinical trials, according to a statement made by the director of the FDA's Oncology Center of Excellence two years later.

- Improvements in Cancer Treatment

In the past, chemotherapy—which employs medications to destroy cancer cells and reduce tumor size—or traditional surgery approaches have been used to treat cancer patients. Thanks to advancements made in clinical trials and experimentation, cancer patients today have access to a variety of cutting-edge therapies.

- New Advances in Alternative Cancer Treatment

Cancer can be treated biologically with immunotherapy, which uses compounds derived from living things. Immune checkpoint inhibitors, monoclonal antibodies, T-cell transfer therapy, vaccinations, and immune system modulators are a few examples of immunotherapy types.

Utilizing the immune system's strength, immunotherapy precisely targets cancer cells while guarding against damage to healthy cells. It can, however, result in adverse effects like fever, chills, weight gain, and heart palpitations.

Drugs that kill cancer cells are activated by light in photodynamic treatment. Photodynamic therapy is a viable alternative for people with skin malignancies and precancers because it doesn't significantly harm healthy cells like other cancer treatments do.

However, this medication has the potential to destroy healthy cells, result in transient photosensitivity, and produce other adverse effects such trouble swallowing, stomach pain, shortness of breath, and skin issues.

Hyperthermia/laser therapy is another complementary cancer treatment that employs light to heat and kill tiny tumors and precancerous cells.

In contrast to surgery, this method of treatment spares the surrounding tissues from harm, takes less time, and has fewer adverse effects like bleeding, pain, infections, and scarring. If safety procedures are not taken, it could pose health hazards.

Targeted therapy uses monoclonal antibodies or small-molecule medicines that can adhere to particular regions of cancer cells to deliver precision medicine. It can assault cancer cells while sparing healthy cells from harm, but it can also result in

Chapter 8:

• Getting Ready for Cancer

Getting Ready for Treatment
Radiation, chemotherapy, and surgery are currently the most often used cancer treatments. One or a combination of these treatments, as well as others, may be given to a cancer patient. The type and stage of your cancer will determine the type of treatment you receive.

• Angels of Imerman

Imerman Angels carefully pairs a cancer survivor (a Mentor Angel) with a person who has been affected by the disease. Additionally, customized matches are made available for

The best strategies to get ready for your treatment sessions should be discussed with your medical team. See if you require laboratory work. Your

Your healthcare professional might offer you advice or write you a prescription for medicine that can help you prevent side effects like nausea.

- Create a medical supply bag.

Many cancer sufferers prepare a specific backpack or tote to bring to their appointments. Include comfort and entertainment things during the duration of treatment, such as:

sweater and relaxed attire.
headphones, a music player, and your favorite songs.
- Pillow and blanket.
- resources for reading.
- activities like crossword puzzles or others.
- playing cards.
- A lip balm.
- lotion for the body.
- peppermint teas, which are calming.

Pen, notebook, and paper.

sock boots.

goodies like cookies or crackers.

the stress ball.

common side effects of treatment

There are side effects to certain treatments. It can make you feel more in control to be aware of what you might go through. Discuss any potential side effects with your medical staff.

Treatment side effects and complications can frequently be reduced with medical attention. Find out what you should not eat or drink while receiving treatment. Additionally, Chemocare.com offers details on how to deal with the side effects of chemotherapy medications.

The three most popular cancer therapy options are described below, along with some potential adverse effects.

- Surgery

Now, improved surgical techniques aid in limiting harm to healthy tissue. Additionally, risks and negative consequences have decreased. Surgery is frequently utilized, such as with a biopsy, to determine the presence of cancer cells.

Tumors can also be removed with it. Surgery may be performed to reconstruct or reshape bodily alterations. Surgery may be used to implant a medical device (port) under the skin. Medication can be administered through the port.

Possible complications following surgery:

- Scarring.

Motion restrictions.
being unable to perform some things permanently or temporarily.
changes to fertility or sexual function.
changes in judgment, learning, or memory (for example, following brain surgery).
Fatigue.

lymphedema or swollenness.
Chemotherapy

Chemotherapy employs drugs to kill cells and halt cell division. These medications can be administered orally as tablets. They can also be administered intravenously (with an IV) or through a port. The drugs circulate throughout the body after entering the bloodstream.

Because the medications target both malignant and non-cancerous cells, side effects do arise. When healthy cells are harmed, negative outcomes can happen.

Chemotherapy is administered in cycles to give the body time to heal in between treatments. Chemotherapy side effects could result from high doses or repeated treatments. Many medications disrupt the body's quickly proliferating cells. These cells may be found in the bone marrow, stomach and intestinal lining, hair, skin, and nails.

Before receiving chemotherapy, discuss potential side effects with your medical team. Treatments for chemotherapy can make you feel sick to your stomach.

Inquire with your doctor about any possible relief from nausea drugs. Some patients advise against consuming your preferred foods immediately before or after therapy. You might not feel like eating those things again later, when it's crucial to recover your appetite and weight.

If you plan to have kids in the future, discuss it with your doctor. If you or your partner think you might be pregnant, be sure to tell your healthcare professional. Chemotherapy can be harmful to a developing youngster.

Cancer patients and survivors whose medical treatments carry the risk of infertility can find reproductive information, support, and hope through Livestrong Fertility.

Costs associated with fertility preservation might be decreased using Livestrong Fertility.

- Possible chemo side effects

Anemia.
- Immunity is reduced.
- Fatigue.
- mouth ulcers.
- Forgetfulness.
- vomiting or nauseous.
- hair fall.
- Raised skin.
- blood and bruises.
- Cataracts.

Following chemotherapy: Everyone is affected by chemotherapy differently. While some have fewer adverse effects than others, others do. The degree to which a treatment is functioning is unrelated to its side effects.

As healthy tissues begin to repair themselves, side effects typically start to get better or disappear. Three weeks after the treatment, this can begin. Even before the therapy is finished, hair can begin to come back.

Concentration may momentarily suffer with chemotherapy. Possible outcomes include slight amnesia. This is also known as "chemo brain" or "chemo fog." Calendars, lists, and voice mail messages can be useful if something occurs to you.

Always share any side effects of chemotherapy with your doctor, such as extreme fatigue, bleeding, numbness and tingling in the limbs (neuropathy), difficulty breathing, issues with eating or drinking, issues with urination or bowel movements, memory loss, difficulty concentrating, pain, infection, and fever.

- radiation treatment

The use of X-rays to a tumor is known as radiation treatment. This could be carried out either internally or topically (on the skin's surface). They could be high or low doses. They are not equivalent to the X-rays used to photograph a tumor.

Vital organs are shielded with lead during therapy. As a result, the radiation harm to healthy tissues around the malignancy is reduced. Additionally, it aids in consistently targeting the same area for treatment.

Radiation side effects can harm the body's healthy cells or structures. During treatment, the doctor will make an effort to avoid exposing nearby tissue to excessive radiation.

To ensure that all cancer is treated, however, some healthy tissue and organs may be affected.

If you intend to have children in the future, discuss this with your doctor before radiation treatment. Prior to beginning radiation therapy, decisions about fertility preservation strategies should be made.

Radiation exposure could harm a fetus, thus women should inform the medical staff if they think they could be pregnant.

Discuss the potential adverse effects of radiation therapy for your particular kind of cancer with your doctor.

Any side effects should be reported as soon as possible to your provider after treatment. Early medical intervention for adverse effects is crucial.

- Head radiation side effects that could occur include:
- Hair changes and hair loss.
- Earaches.
- mouth irritation and redness.
- dry mouth, swallowing issues, or taste alterations.
- changes to the mouth, throat, teeth, or gums.
- Radiation may have adverse consequences on the body.

- Children who are still growing experience changes in bone development.
- Skin that is dry, irritable, or red.
- diarrhea, vomiting, or nausea.
- digestion and eating issues.
- bladder irritability.
- effects on sexual function or fertility.

- Breast size fluctuates
- Fibrosis (scarring or stiffness) of the lungs.
- bone thinning or osteoporosis.
- Radiation side effects in general
- weakness or drowsiness.
- Soreness and swelling.
- coughing or breathing difficulties.
- Low quantities of platelets or white blood cells (rare).
- effects on the heart.

A treatment called hormone therapy involves adding, blocking, or removing hormones. Surgery may be required with this form of treatment to remove a gland that produces a specific hormone.

Hormones may be administered in various circumstances to raise low hormone levels. In order to delay or stop the growth of some malignancies, synthetic hormones or other medications may be used to disrupt the body's natural hormones.

Prostate and breast cancer may be treated in this way. The advantages and hazards of this kind of medication, such as osteoporosis, should be discussed with your healthcare professional.

Treatment for Cancer and Fatigue
Observe What Takes Place Between Medical Appointments

One of the most typical adverse effects of cancer treatment is fatigue or feeling physically weary. It's possible that you won't have the energy to accomplish your priorities. You may experience mental and emotional effects from fatigue.

Physical issues including pain, stress, anemia, or medication side effects are some examples of the reasons for weariness. Sometimes the root of the problem is emotional, like depression. Sometimes the root issue might not be obvious. However, weariness is typically successfully treated medically.

If you feel worn out, let your healthcare professional know. Use phrases like light, moderate, or severe to describe your level of exhaustion. In order to offer the best treatment to help relieve the weariness, your medical team will work to determine what is causing it.

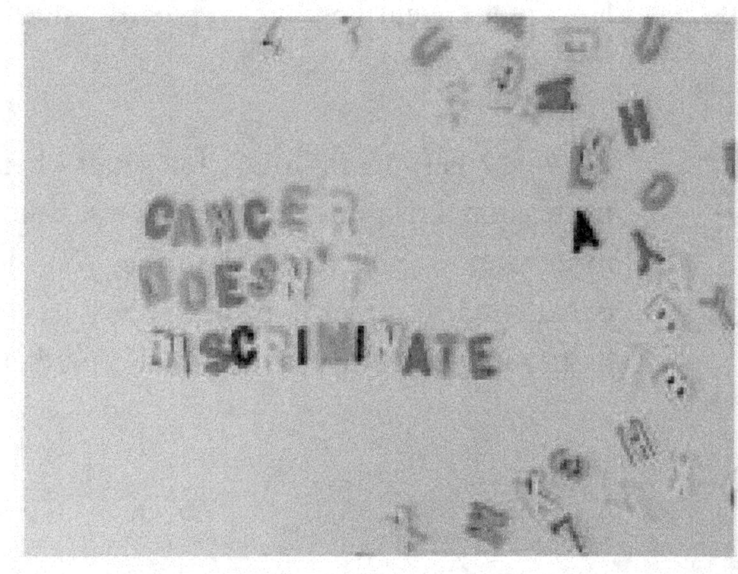

Chapter 9:

Which medical procedures are worthwhile?

useful in reducing pain in cancer cases. Also, it might ease stress, weariness, and anxiety. Still, massage can be safe, If you work with a professed massage therapist.

numerous cancer treatment installations have massage therapists on staff, or your croaker can recommend a massage therapist who constantly treats cancer cases.

still, avoid getting a massage, If you have extremely low blood counts. Request that the massage therapist chorus from working on or near any excrescences, radiation treatment spots, or surgical scars.

Ask the massage therapist to use light pressure rather than deep massage if you have osteoporosis, cancer of the bones, or any other bone problems. Contemplation. When you concentrate your mind on a single image, sound, or idea, similar to a positive study, you're in a profound position of attention.

You might also exercise deep breathing or relaxation ways while planning. Contemplation may profit cancer cases by reducing stress and anxiety and elevating mood.

In general, contemplation is secure. You can either do a class with an educator or meditate on your own for a many twinkles formerly or doubly per day. Also, there are a ton of guided contemplation operations and online courses accessible.

music treatment. You might sing, play an instrument, or produce lyrics while sharing in music remedy sessions.

You can take part in music remedy in a group setting or under the guidance of a good music therapist who'll guide you through conditioning provisioned to your unique requirements.

As well as decreasing torment, concern, and tension, music cure may likewise prop with queasiness and choking activity.

Music gift isn't important to participate in music cure, which is protected. dinkum
Music specialists work in a ton of medical clinics. ways for unwinding.

practicing unwinding ways will assist you with focusing on decreasing pressure and progressing your body.
Moderate strong unwinding and perception practices are two examples of unwinding ways.

Tension and exhaustion might be diminished with the guide of unwinding ways. Ways for unwinding are secure. These activities are for the most part directed by a specialist, however at last you might be reasonable to perform them freely or with the guide of directed unwinding accounts.

Chi gung. Judo is a type of activity that joins slow, purposeful breathing with delicate developments.

You can learn judo with an educator, or you can do it single-handedly by watching or perusing books regarding the matter.

Kendo activities could diminish pressure. Judo is basically inconvenience free. Since judo moves gradually, it doesn't require a great deal of actual strength, and the schedules are easy to change to your own capacities.

In any case, counsel your croaker prior to beginning judo. Keep away from any agonizing tai ki developments. Yoga. Yoga blends profound taking in with extending works out. You orchestrate your body in various stances during a yoga meeting that call for bowing, winding, and extending. Yoga arrives in different structures, each with novel variations.

Individuals with malignant growth might discover some relief from stress through yoga. Additionally demonstrated to upgrade rest and decrease exhaustion is yoga.

Prior to signing up for a yoga class, request your croaker for the name from a yoga preceptor who has experience working with visitors who have issues, practically equivalent to a disease.

Keep away from any excruciating yoga positions. A brilliant preceptor can give safe druthers for your positions.

A few operations could cycle each other successfully. For case, profound breathing while at the same time entering a back rub could assist with lessening pressure to be sure further.

Chapter 10:

1. Life Past Disease Figuring out Endurance

As well as decreasing torment, concern, and tension, music cure may likewise prop with queasiness and choking activity.
Music gift isn't important to participate in music cure, which is protected. dinkum
Music specialists work in a ton of medical clinics.

ways for unwinding. Practicing unwinding ways will assist you with focusing on decreasing pressure and progressing your body.

Moderate strong unwinding and perception practices are two examples of unwinding ways.

Tension and exhaustion might be diminished with the guide of unwinding ways. Ways for unwinding are secure.

These activities are for the most part directed by a specialist, however at last you might be reasonable to perform them freely or with the guide of directed unwinding accounts. Chi gung. Judo is a type of activity that joins slow, purposeful breathing with delicate developments.

You can learn judo with an educator, or you can do it single-handedly by watching or perusing books regarding the matter.

Kendo activities could diminish pressure. Judo is basically inconvenience free. Since judo moves gradually, it doesn't request a great deal of actual strength, and the schedules are easy to change to your own capacities. in any case, counsel your croaker prior to beginning judo.

Keep away from any agonizing tai ki developments. Yoga. Yoga blends profound taking in with extending works out. You orchestrate your body in various stances during a yoga meeting that call for bowing, winding, and extending.

Yoga arrives in different structures, each with novel variations. Individuals with malignant growth might discover some relief from stress through yoga.

Additionally demonstrated to upgrade rest and decrease exhaustion is yoga.

Prior to signing up for a yoga class, request your croaker for the name from a yoga preceptor who has experience working with visitors who have issues, practically equivalent to a disease.

Keep away from any excruciating yoga positions. A brilliant preceptor can give safe druthers for your positions.

A few operations could cycle each other successfully. For case, profound breathing while at the same time entering a back rub could assist with lessening pressure to be sure further.

2. Perceiving Endurance

Figures on disease survivorship

Bosom, lung, colorectal, and prostate disease endurance rates at one and five years for the

WCRF network countries (the Netherlands, the UK, and the US).

For what reason do disease endurance rates vary between countries?

Following a disease finding, endurance is impacted by various elements.

The most continuous factors incorporate the sort of malignant growth recognized, the medicines that can be utilized, and the phase of the infection when it is found and when treatment starts.

As a general rule, improved results and endurance are connected to before malignant growth ID.

The pervasiveness of a few site-explicit malignancies has expanded throughout the course of recent many years because of enhancements in screening projects and treatments.

There are contrasts in admittance to medical care inside nations, and medical services frameworks differ among countries.

Contrasts in endurance rates are impacted by the two components. Lower pay nations normally have lower endurance rates, while there is huge change among top level salary nations.

Research on the associations between diet, sustenance, and actual work and disease endurance is extending.

We discovered some, though restricted, proof that keeping a sound weight, participating in normal active work, and sticking to a solid eating regimen (especially eating food sources wealthy in fiber and soy and devouring less immersed fat) may further develop endurance after bosom malignant growth.

Our Worldwide Disease Update Program is the world's biggest wellspring of logical examination on malignant growth avoidance and survivorship through diet, nourishment, and actual work.

To give suggestions on diet, nourishment, and actual work for endurance from extra site-explicit malignancies and disease by and large, more examination is required.

After a malignant growth conclusion and after the intense phase of therapy

(during which a patient should consent to their essential consideration doctor's dietary suggestions), we exhorted following our malignant growth counteraction proposals since they may likewise assist with forestalling other non-transmittable infections (like cardiovascular sickness and type 2 diabetes).

For what reason are malignant growth explicit endurance rates unique?

As well as being affected by the phase of location, conclusion, and treatment, endurance rates vary by sort of disease.

For example, as indicated by the latest information from the UK, the level of bosom disease patients who are as yet alive five years after their finding is more than 80%.

Be that as it may, the 5-year endurance rate for certain growths, such cellular breakdown in the lungs, is under 20%.

The way that more people with different malignant growth types had before analyzed accounts to some extent for higher endurance rates.

This may be because of screening programs being offered and utilized, which brings about prior revelation and conclusion.

An individual's wellbeing, the pervasiveness of comorbid conditions, and other growth related variables can all influence endurance.

Rather than other malignant growth sorts, some disease structures keep on being trying to analyze or potentially treat notwithstanding progressions in study and innovation.

- Meanings of endurance rate

The level of malignant growth patients who are as yet alive one year after their determination or the beginning of treatment is known as the 1-year endurance rate.

The level of malignant growth patients who are as yet alive five years after their determination or the start of treatment is known as the 5-year endurance rate.

Conclusion:

The Future-Free Toolkit

COLLABORATING TO BUILD A HEALTHY
FUTURE

This past year, we were able to make a
difference in communities around Illinois and
beyond because to your contributions. Together,
we overcame fresh obstacles, developed fresh
answers, and advanced the cause of a world
without lung disease.

We want to highlight some of our efforts to
prevent lung disease, promote clean air, and
improve the quality of life for those who already
have lung disease as we approach the end of our
program year.

- ASTHMA

We created a new resource in collaboration with the Illinois Network of Child Care Resource and Referral Agencies (INCCRRA) for childcare providers all throughout the state to assist children in their care who have asthma. The English or Spanish versions have been viewed by more than 2,500 individuals since their debut.

- ENVIRONMENT

The Climate and Equitable Jobs Act (CEJA), a pioneering equitable climate law in the country, was passed after three years of activism and leadership with numerous partner groups.

We continue to take the lead in carrying out these initiatives, especially when it comes to working with legislators to hasten the electrification of transportation in the entire state. The CEJA puts Illinois on the path to use only renewable energy by the year 2050.

- ## CONDUCT OF AIR

We are spearheading a coalition to achieve the adoption of Advanced Clean Truck regulations in response to a recent investigation that found significant health hazards from diesel pollution in Illinois.

By electrifying heavy-duty trucks, this initiative, made possible by funding from the Energy Foundation, will lessen the dangers posed by diesel emissions today.

- ## THROAT CANCER

We collaborated with healthcare partners to identify barriers to these screenings in Illinois in order to increase access to lung cancer tests for high-risk individuals.

Together, we were successful in securing$ 1 million in backing in Illinois to support educating the public about and exercising these services.

Adding access to these precautionary treatments will promote the early discovery of lung cancer in those who are most at threat, maybe saving lives.

COVID- 19 We're starting a new trouble to produce case- facing coffers concerning the implicit goods of extended COVID thanks to an entitlement from the Will Rogers Institute.

We'll be in the van of spreading mindfulness about these new problems and aiding those who are most vulnerable to maintain their health as new exploration continues to show the long-term impacts of habitual COVID.

COPD It might be grueling to give to a friend or family member who has COPD. According to estimates, 16 million individuals worldwide have COPD, and millions more experience symptoms but warrant an opinion.

This demonstrates the increased demand for caregiver support among the COPD community. with the backing of the National Heart, Lung, and Blood Institute.

moment, informal caregivers each over the nation have easier access to services to help them deal with the difficulties of minding for their loved bones

Health of women's lungs Our Catch Your Breath ® women's lung health crusade has grown remarkably, and we're continuing to spread mindfulness of the unique hazards that lung complaints pose for women.

We were fortunate to work with the CHEST Foundation formerly more this time to support promising exploration examining differences in women's lung health.

Together with the Illinois Health Practice Alliance, a provider of internal health services with further than 100 conventions in Illinois that accept Medicaid cases, exploration To support fresh disquisition into lung cancer, idiopathic pulmonary fibrosis(IPF), and COPD, we handled finances. In order to more target and enhance cancer treatments, one ofDr.

Maria Lucia Madariaga's examinations on lung cancer examines new styles for examining lung towels.

The University of Washington'sDr. Laura Feemster's work on COPD exploration was supported by our periodic Solovy Award for Advancement in COPD.

Learn further about the exploration, policy, and educational enterprise that your donations fund.

You can also subscribe up for updates on our sweats to ensure that everyone has access to clean air and healthy lungs.

still, promote clean air, and aid those who formerly have lung illness, If you want to help the RHA avoid lung complaints.